The Easy Vegan Beginners Guide

Boosts Your Energy & Improves Health

Written By
Julie Sobers

Disclaimer

The material in this book is for general guidance and the author assumes no liability for the consequences of its misuse, loss or expense incurred as a result of relying on the information in this book.

Social Media

Instagram: JulietheVegan

Twitter: @JulietheVegan

Facebook: Julie the Vegan

Youtube: Julie the Vegan

Website: www.juliethevegan.org

Contents

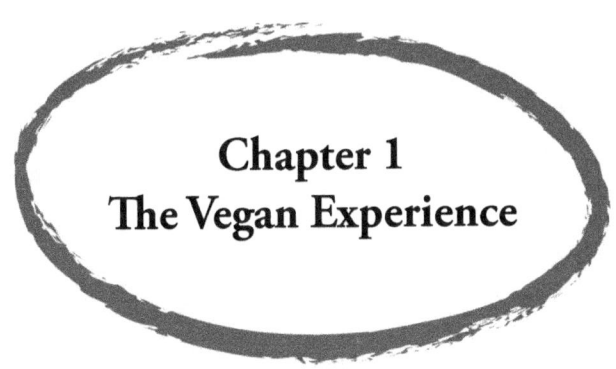

Chapter 1
The Vegan Experience

1. The Vegan Experience

Welcome, Congratulations and a Big Hug!!

If you are reading this book because you want to try out the vegan diet or you are already a vegan but want some extra tips you are making a choice which has the potential to greatly improve your life.

To be honest with you I never had any interest in understanding what a vegan was nor did I want to be a vegan. But now, my journey of becoming a vegan and embracing the vegan lifestyle has changed my life in so many great ways and I want to be able to share my experience and steps I took to become vegan to make sure that you can start your vegan diet the easy way. I am Julie the Vegan and I am here for you because I care.

How to Go Vegan the Easy Way

Thank you for at least entertaining the possibility of being a vegan and being open to the concept. Before you read this entire book I'm sure you would like to dive straight into finding out why it's easy to be a vegan? Are you ready? Stop buying animal products. Finito!

It literally is that simple, no tests need to be taken, you don't need to live in a particular country or buy any fancy kitchen equipment, and you don't even need to finish reading the rest of this book. For some people they become vegan over night for other people they transition gradually into the vegan diet.

My Vegan Experience

For many years I had suffered from anemia and my solutions were iron supplements and coffee. I really enjoyed drinking coffee because of the effect it had on giving me that boost of energy in the morning and transforming me from a zombie into a functional human and I found myself dependent on coffee to help me retain my high energetic state.

Coffee definitely helped me get through my days and I very much enjoyed drinking it, however, the regularity of my coffee intake would result in me experiencing heart palpitations, my hands would shake and I would get severe headaches. My body was very sensitive to the caffeine and my body couldn't cope with it in my system. Coffee is also very dehydrating and I would experience regular headaches which I would mask with paracetamol to take the pain of it away.

You can only imagine the combination of all the coffee and numbing paracetamol medication in my system caused me to loose all connection with my body and I was unable to hear my body telling me that it was getting very ill because it was intoxicated as a result of the choices I was making to drink coffee. So the only thing my body could do to get my attention was to shut down and make me feel extreme pain and discomfort.

At that time in my life I was a university student and it was the morning of a very important university examination and I awoke to find myself experiencing hot and cold flushes, I was dizzy and was very ill, my body was shutting down. In that morning I literally thought that was the end for me.

My doctor told me the symptoms I was experiencing were related to my body being very sensitive to the caffeine in coffee, I was dehydrated and that is why it and such a profound impact on my health. I wanted to be able to feel my body again and listen to what it likes and what it doesn't like because I wanted to regain control of my health. So from that moment on I made the decision stop drinking anything containing caffeine and said goodbye to my beloved coffee.

When I stopped drinking coffee I needed to find natural alternatives for me to elevate and sustain my energy levels. So I started to research natural alternatives to coffee using books and the internet to find a solution.

The first thing I found was eliminating red meat from the diet because it takes the body a lot of time and energy to break down meat in the body. By eliminating meat you can conserve a lot more of your energy. So I did a little experiment on myself I stopped eating meat and within 2 days I had a lot more energy.

So I searched for other solutions and came across green juices. So, I bought myself a juicer and the first green juice I ever drank gave me the same effects as having an espresso. It was such an exciting experience to know that there were natural alternatives to coffee and all I had to do was just find them.

As of that point I had eliminated all red meats and coffee, but I was still eating chicken, fish and dairy products. But because I had experienced such great results from removing meat from my diet I decided to remove chicken also, then a few months later I removed fish, but still continued to eat dairy. I still had no interest in becoming a vegan I just new I was feeling better and healthier and that was good enough for me.

My health was going from strength to strength and I came to the understanding that I was a vegetarian. Not only was I a vegetarian but I was becoming more and more interested in veganism, however, I was finding it very difficult to stop eating dairy products. All that changed when I became more aware of the animal cruelty aspects of not being a vegan and that was definitely an extra motivating factor to help me stop eating dairy and keep me vegan. Because it wasn't just good for me but also great for our fellow animal friends and also the planet. So all in all a win, win for all and everything. So I then went 100% vegan!!

Since becoming 100% vegan I have noticed that I no longer need to use my iron supplements because my anemia is now under control and I have more energy than ever before. My acne has cleared up, my nails and hair started to grow long and strong. I was experiencing so many amazing benefits that I just wanted to continue and see what other amazing benefits were in store for me to experience.

As of now I am a raw vegan which consists of obtaining the majority of my calories from fresh raw fruit and vegetables. I feel even more amazing, so much happier and look forward to what the future holds.

Chapter 2
Its All About You

2. Its All About You

What is a Vegan Diet?

Consists of all food with the exception of animal products. A healthy vegan diet is a plant based diet.

Your Why?

You need to find out and establish your why you want to ditch meat and dairy because that is the only reason why you will start and stay a vegan.

If you ask 100 vegans why they do not consume any animal products you may receive 100 different answers. But of all the reasons there are 3 in general which are always at the top of the list.

- Personal health
- Animal suffering
- Concern for the Environment

Personal Health

The health advantages of a plant-based diet are endless. Both British and American Dietetic Association also medical research affirm that a well-planned plant based vegan diet prevents many ailments, helps reverse some, and eases the symptoms of others to support healthy living at every age.

The biggest and fastest growing health epidemic is obesity. It is estimated that more than 500 million people suffer from obesity worldwide today and kills more than 3 million people each year. The leading cause of death in the world today is heart disease and the cause of 7million deaths a year. These are very serious problems with a very simple solution.

A plant based diet is low in saturated fat, high in fiber and packed with antioxidants, which helps prevent the vast majority of life threatening diseases that plague modernity.

More advantages include significantly reduced rates of hypertension, arterial hardening, stroke, type 2 diabetes, obesity, heart disease and several types of cancer (prostate and breast cancer are the most documented).

A plant based vegan diet is naturally cholesterol free, and is almost guaranteed to lead to marked decreases in cholesterol levels in just 2 weeks. Blood pressure too is shown to decrease drastically in a short period of time on a plant based diet.

Animal Suffering

All of the protein, iron, calcium, vitamins and minerals the human body requires can be obtained on a plant based vegan diet. Why not just cut out the middle man and get the vitamins and nutrients our body needs straight from the source in an ethical way.

All living animals fear death, just as much as we do. And animals feel pain just as much as we do. Ethically a vegan diet makes sense. If you had a pet dog would you one day decide to kill it and eat it? Highly unlikely because ethically you could not justify your actions. The exact same principle applies to all animals.

If you had to slaughter animals by hand every time you ate some meat or chicken you probably would not want to eat it. But going to the supermarket and buying it in a packet desensitises us from understanding what exactly happened to that animal before it was on the shelf in the store. The slaughter, torture and torment that animal had to endure for the consumption by man is entirely unnecessary because we have plenty of alternatives which are healthier for us and in addition a lot more ethical. Man doesn't need to eat the flesh of an animal to survive and live.

Environmental Damage

Raising animals for food requires massive amounts of land, food, energy and water. The by-products of animal agriculture pollute our air and waterways. It's time to think of waste as well as taste.

The way we breed animals is now recognised by the UN, scientists, economists and politicians as giving rise to many interlinked human and ecological problems, but with 1 billion people already not having enough to eat and 3 billion more mouths to feed within 50 years, the urgency to rethink our relationship with animals is extreme because the alternative of doing nothing and turning a blind eye is just not good enough anymore and doesn't bear thinking about.

- **Polluting the air**

  The transport and other processes involved from farm to fork places a heavy burden on the environment. Carbon dioxide, methane and nitrous oxide combined cause the vast majority of global warming.

From recycling our household waste to cycling to work, we're all aware of ways to live a greener life. Did you know removing meat and dairy from your diet is the simplest and cheapest way to reduce your carbon footprint and reduce human impact on the environment.

- **Polluting the water**

Each day, factory farms produce billions of pounds of waste, manure, nitrogen compounds and fertilizers which end up in lakes, rivers, oceans and drinking water. This pollution causes algal blooms which take up all the oxygen in the water to the point where little can live in that environment and is also contaminating drinking water.

- **Using up land resources**

As the worlds appetite for meat increases, countries across the globe are bulldozing huge swaths of land to make more room for animals, also the crops and grain required to feed them. This is a significant contributor to deforestation, habitat loss and species extinction.

The sheer quantity of animals now being raised for humans to eat now threatens the earth's biodiversity. A plant based diet requires only one third of the land needed to support a meat and dairy diet.

- **Using up drinking water resources**

  Farming uses 70% of water available to humans and is already in direct competition for water with cities. Rich but water stressed countries such as Saudi Arabia, Libya, Gulf states and South Africa all say it makes sense to grow food in poorer countries to conserve their water resources, and are now buying or leasing millions of hectares of Ethiopia and elsewhere to provide their food.

  Every cow fattened in Gambella state in southern Ethiopia is exported to Abu Dhabi or Britain. This is taking the pressure of water supplies back home, but increasing it elsewhere.

  With rising global food and water insecurity due to the ever increasing world population and global warming, there's never been a better time to adopt a more sustainable way of living–and avoiding animal products is one of the simplest ways to start.

Chapter 3
Why Being Vegetarian is Not Good Enough

3. Why Being Vegetarian is Not Good Enough

Do you know what is in your milk and cheese? Dairy contains puss, bacteria and viruses. Our deeply rooted beliefs about the wholesomeness of milk and dairy products needs to be reconsidered.

Puss

Legally 135 million puss cells are allowed in one glass of milk. Puss cells also known as somatic cells are the same type of cells produced from a giant spot on your forehead. The puss cells in cows are produced as a result of infected udders. This is essentially the same liquid that is released when you pop a spot on your face. So that same puss is what you drink in your milk.

Synthetic Growth Hormones

Synthetic hormones such as recombinant bovine growth hormone (rGBH) are pumped into animals producing dairy to increase their milk production but can imbalance human hormones because it interferes with our sensitive endocrine regularity network from the fetal period into old age and triggers the growth of cancer.

Osteoporosis

Bones are designed to last a lifetime. They should remain strong. So we must be living by the wrong set of rules to cause a disease such as Osteoporosis. From a young age we have been conditioned that we need milk for healthy strong bones. However, there has been no research study which shows drinking milk reduces the risk of fractures. But research has shown that drinking milk actually increases your risk of bone fractures by 50%.

Milk Protein

The main protein in milk is called 'Casein' and is toxic for humans. It is directly responsible for:, Eczema, Acne, Kidney disease, Arthritis, Tooth Decay, Asthma, Irritable bowles, Sinus problems, Colitis, Crohn's, MS, and especially breast and prostate cancer.

Natural Animal Hormones

Just as humans have hormones in their milk which are beneficial for babies, cows have hormones in their milk beneficial for their calves. Cow's milk contains over 80 active hormones which are not meant to be in the human body thus can cause a whole host of problems.

When those active hormones enter our human body, our entire body goes into complete inflammation because our bodies don't understand what these hormones are. There is one hormone called IGF -1 and when it's taken into the human body it makes our pituitary gland secrete more growth hormone. So if you have cancer that causes more cells to replicate. But also people are often unaware they have cancer until it gets to a size which causes concern, so prevention is always better than cure

Ethical Dairy and Eggs

Male chicks are worthless to the egg and meat industry because they will not lay eggs and will not grow large enough or fast enough for meat, so are killed. Male calves suffer the same fate because they do not produce milk so are just as worthless to dairy farms and are also killed just because of their gender. Cows can live 15 years on average but are slaughtered prematurely when their milk production decreases which is usually after 4 years. Eating dairy and eggs supports this treatment of animals.

Chapter 4
The Vegan Diet Journey

4. The Vegan Diet Journey

Break Old Habits

If you're used to eating eggs for breakfast, chicken for lunch and steak for dinner you may be wondering what's left? As a matter of habit, most people reach for the same few foods day after day. But there are nearly an infinite array of fresh fruit, vegetables, beans, legumes, grains and herbs from all around the world at your fingertips.

All you have to do is get creative and the vegan diet will bring even more flavors, color and variety to your plate than ever before.

Additive

It's actually much easier and simpler to focus on what vegans can eat instead of what vegans do not eat. This shift in focus will enable you to fully embrace the vegan diet and make it easier for you to eat food you enjoy.

With the addition of food alternatives, more fresh fruits and vegetables all your taste and nutritional needs will be met as a vegan.

There is No Vegan Contract

There is no right way to become a vegan but there are ways to make it easier for yourself, if it is something that you do want to do. If you want to be a vegan, you will be a vegan. Your journey can be as long or as short as you want it to be. There is no contract to being a vegan it is all within your control and you can do whatever you want.

There is no rush so there is no need to force yourself, or make yourself feel unhappy by applying pressure to yourself. Just do your best and that is good enough.

Setbacks are Normal

If you slip up and have a glass of milk, or eat some chicken wings that doesn't mean that you can no longer be vegan. Just always be aware and conscious of the food choices you make and continue right back on with your vegan experience. Nobody is perfect. Your vegan diet can last a lifetime or it can last a week or a few months. Don't beat yourself up about it if you slip back into old eating habits because eventually you will become 100% vegan and be able to sustain that dietary choice.

Chapter 5
What Can You Eat
as a Vegan?

5. What Can You Eat as a Vegan?

What Can You Eat as a Vegan

The vegan diet is a plant based diet and vegans mostly eat whole foods (fruits, vegetables, beans, nuts, seeds, grains) but there are a variety of meat and dairy free substitutes for traditional favorites (burgers, pizza, ice cream) which can be found in most supermarkets. So you have the option to still eat all your familiar food using the vegan version.

There are many health benefits of a vegan diet but not all vegan food is healthy such as french fries and crisps. So when it comes to vegan nutrition variety of healthy choices is key to maintain a balanced diet.

Vegan and Raw Vegan Cuisine

Incorporating lots of fresh raw living fruit and veg into your diet will allow for the vitamins, minerals and nutrients in the food to be available for the body to absorb and use efficiently and effectively. Cooking fresh fruit or vegetables destroys the vitamins, minerals and nutrients and the food is not as healthy to eat.

Raw vegan food has living enzymes which help break down and digest the food in your body so your body will not need to use an excess of energy to digest food. However, when the food is cooked the enzymes are denatured so your body needs to use energy to digest the food which is often the reason why you can feel sleepy after eating a cooked meal.

Some Vegan Food Alternatives

Very often the most common food which people find difficult to find alternatives for is dairy, but there are lots of foods which you can use as alternatives to dairy. Milk, cheese and butter alternatives are high in fat and should be eaten in moderation to maintain a healthy balanced diet.

Milk alternatives:

- Coconut milk

- Almond milk

- Rice milk

Cheese alternatives:

- Nutritional yeast

- Vegan cheese

- Avocado

- Hummus

Butter alternatives:

- Almond butter

- Coconut butter

Meat chicken and fish usually have a place on your plate for every meal. Alternatives to meat, chicken and fish include:

- Beans and pulses
- Tofu
- Vegetables
- Quinoa
- Lentils

Doesn't Have to be Bland

Incorporating a variety of flavors will make meals very enjoyable. Vegan food does not have to be bland as you can use seasoning, spices and sauces on your food. Also, buying fresh organic fruit and vegetables have a lot more flavor than non-organic produce.

Organic

No genetically modified organisms (GMO), no harsh chemicals or preservatives which can all cause illness and allergies.

Vegan Whilst Travelling

You will need to be prepared. You can bring fresh fruit or dried fruit, vegetable snacks or even fresh smoothies and juices are all delicious and easy to travel with. You cannot expect other people to cater for you in this society as it is now. So you will need to be independent in your food choices and prepare food yourself. At least you know what's in it and you will not go hungry.

Chapter 6
Where Will I Get
My Protein?

6. Where Will I Get My Protein?

One of the most common questions and concerns people have about the vegan diet is 'Where will I get my protein from?'. But that question will be answered right now along with other answers to common questions relative to nutrient and vitamin sources for vegans.

Where Will You Get Your Protein From?

Despite the obsession with protein, majority of people eat far too much protein than is recommended and deficiencies in vegans is pretty much unheard of.

All fruit and vegetables contain protein but foods which have high levels of protein include:

- Hemp seeds
- Spiralina
- beans and pulses
- quinoa
- Nuts and seeds
- Brown rice
- Peas

Make sure your protein sources are varied, rather than just from one food group.

The Vegan Diet is Dairy Free So Where Will You Get Your Calcium?

- Dark leafy green vegetables
- Spinach

- Broccoli
- Almonds

Where Will You Get Your Vitamin D?

The vegan diet does not readily supply vitamin D which is an important nutrient. However, vitamin D is very easily obtained from sunlight.

- Just step outside for a few minutes every day and your set with vitamin D

Where Will You Get Your B12?

B12 cannot reliably be obtained from vegan foods. Long term vegans and pregnant and breast-feeding women in particular need a reliable source.

- Take a supplement
- Fortified foods such as nutritional yeast

Where Will You Get Your Omega 3 Fatty Acids?

Fish Oils and fish such as salmon and mackerel are often the most common sources people will eat for their source of omega-3 fatty acids. The vegan sources of omega - 3 fatty acids include:

- Flax seeds
- Flax oil
- Hemp seeds
- Walnuts

Where Will You Get Your Iron?

Vegans actually get a lot more iron in their diet than omnivores because the basis of a vegan diet is plant based. The sources of food with high iron levels are:

- Dark leafy green vegetables

- Kale

- Spinach

- Lentils

- Chickpeas

- Tahini

When it comes to vegan nutrition, variety is key. Eat a rainbow of fruits and veggies, and include green leafy vegetables as often as possible.

Chapter 7
The Vegan Lifestyle Journey

7. The Vegan Lifestyle Journey

The full expression of being a vegan is not just limited to the diet but incorporates the vegan lifestyle. Becoming a vegan may not necessarily happen overnight it's most definitely a journey. But fully embracing being a vegan will make your vegan diet a lot easier to maintain long term.

Benefits of Adopting a Vegan Lifestyle

The main benefits of adopting a vegan lifestyle include enhanced natural beauty, increased energy levels, increased mental clarity, more spiritually aware, more compassionate and healthier.

The vegan lifestyle will naturally develop the longer you maintain your vegan diet and will make your choice of being a vegan a lot more enjoyable, sustainable and easier.

The Vegan Lifestyle Includes:

- **Drink lots of water**

  The average adult body is 50-65% water so drinking adequate amounts of water will prevent dehydration and allow your body to function effectively and efficiently as it should. Also water helps to detoxify the body and helps to prevent fatigue, pimples and digestive issues.

- **Exercise**

  You will have more energy and feel more motivated to exercise and be out in nature.

Getting the body moving, encouraging the blood to flow around your body will help to ensure you can remain healthy. Exercise also releases endorphins known as 'happy hormones' that help us gain the right mental composure.

- **Sleep**

  Rest and recuperation of the body is important to maintain your health, live longer and research has shown sleep can help with weight issues.

- **Take control of your life**

  Fully embracing being a vegan will allow for you to take control of your diet and in turn you will develop the skills to take control of your life. You can be whoever you want to be and achieve whatever you want to create.

- **More conscious and compassionate**

  When you are more conscious of what you are putting into your body you become more conscious of what you are putting on your body. You will be more conscious about being compassionate with yourself for what you eat, you become more compassionate for the way you look. You will fully embrace and love yourself and in turn will have a lot more compassion and understanding for other people and for animals. Everything you do and say will change when adopting the vegan lifestyle.

- **Enhanced natural beauty**

    You will develop a natural glow as the way you look begins to change. Eating foods which are fresh and living contains lots of highly positive vibrations which can only bring about a feeling of increased happiness and joy which other people will be able to see emanating from you.

Chapter 8
What Has Love Got
To Do With It?

8. What Has Love Got To Do With It?

Now more than ever I have come to the understanding that my vegan experience has nothing to do with me, although it starts with me. But it is for love, love of self, others, animals, planet. Love for all. I now see there never was nor ever shall be a separation or divide when love is present, there is no hierarchy in love. Love has no boundaries and remains victorious in times of doubt.

Connecting with your inner voice, connects you with the truth of all truths which is love. With love all things became clear and our true nature can be found and once found explored, once explored accepted, once accepted expressed, once expressed manifested abundantly with no limits and no separation.

The more I connected with who I was and trusted my inner voice, the more I connected with compassion and love and acceptance of self. I then wanted other people to feel the freedom of self-love and wanted all living creatures to benefit from this freedom also.

I want all people, all animals and our planet to be treated with love, compassion and acceptance. The more I follow my inner voice, the more confirmation presents itself to me in the world that what I am feeling is right and true.

Through god's love for me, that love has helped and allowed me to love myself so I can truly love other people, animals, and our planet. I can love my reflection. For my reflection is me in all aspects of nature, we are all connected we are all one.

My vegan experience is one based in love. Loving myself enough to say I will do whatever it takes to make sure that I am healthy, happy and feel good. Taking an inward focus on self-love, of true feelings and going with the flow of what is the right thing to do, and not following what society has considered the accepted norm after years of excessive propaganda.

Look within to see the truth and do the right thing regardless of any adversity or discouragement. Stay strong and continue on.

Chapter 9
Top 3 Tips To
Stay Motivated

9. Top 3 Tips To Stay Motivated

Remember Your Why

Eating animals contributes to animal cruelty and suffering. Eating animals contributes to making yourself unhealthy and ill. Eating animals you are setting an example to others that it's ok to abuse and destroy our planet. Be the change you want to see in the world. Establish and write down your reason why you started the vegan diet and you will always have your initial purpose to keep you motivated with your choice of embracing veganism.

Have Vegan Friends

Involve yourself in the vegan community so you can meet other people to keep you motivated and encouraged to follow through with your vegan diet. You can ask for help and tips for long term success.

Educate Yourself

Learn new recipes and explore different varieties of fresh fruit and vegetables. Knowledge is power, the more information you know about the vegan diet the better choices you will be able to make to ensure long term success with your vegan diet.

For more information and resources visit:
Website: www.juliethevegan.org